# Connections:

## Activities for Alzheimer's & Dementia Patients

## A Practical Guide for Caregivers and Families

Stacy Lee Andersen

For Chelsea

and

Chance

# Introduction

During my years working in long-term care, I searched and researched endless hours, looking for the perfect activities for Alzheimer's and dementia patients. I was never satisfied with the books on the market.

Some of the books expected that I had access to an endless budget for crafts, games and food--not the case! Other books listed activities that required planning and preparation—however, I found that when dealing with people, whether at home or in a care facility, things never went as planned. Someone had a doctor's appointment, visitors arrived unexpectedly, or residents became ill.

I also wanted a book that focused on the patient. Many times, activity books are written with a "facilitator as leader" approach. However, I felt that the facilitator/caregiver should not be the leader or the center of the activity. I wanted everyone to feel that we were all on the same level. I didn't want to teach or preach. I wanted to learn and explore with the resident.

Through trial and error, I explored my thoughts and ideas with people of various cognitive levels. I wrote this book for all health care workers who, despite the demands of their work, truly aim to make a difference.

# Activity Survey

What are the interests of your loved one or group? Try handing out a sample activity survey to the group. Read the survey aloud, and ask participants to circle items that are most interesting to them. If you type your own version of the survey, keep in mind to use large typeface for those with poor eyesight.

| | | |
|---|---|---|
| Art | TV | Movies |
| Decorating | Food | Cooking |
| History | Poetry | Fiction |
| Biography | Science | Health |
| Board games | Card games | Gardening |
| Animals | Plants | Music |
| Foreign language | Sports | Exercise |

# Who's the Inventor?

Who invented the camera?

    a) Sir Walter, b) George Eastman, Fred Algrove

Who invented Coca-Cola?

    a) Bob Rogers, b) Todd Freeman, c) John Pemberton

Who invented the cotton gin?
    a) Eli Whitney, b) Andy Smith, c) Beth Jones

Who invented dynamite?
    a) Leroy Snout, b) Alfred Nobel, c) Michael Lang

Who invented the phonograph?
    a) Thomas Edison, b) Ernest Black, c) Jack Nepple

Who invented the telephone?
    a) James Hirsch, b) Marcus Devine, c) Alexander Graham Bell

Who invented the revolver?

    a) Leon Dahl, b) Allen White, c) Samuel Colt

*Answers: b, c, a, b, a, c, a, c*

# States and Capitals

| | |
|---|---|
| Alabama | Montgomery |
| Alaska | Juneau |
| Arizona | Phoenix |
| Arkansas | Little Rock |
| California | Sacramento |
| Colorado | Denver |
| Connecticut | Hartford |
| Delaware | Dover |
| Florida | Tallahassee |
| Georgia | Atlanta |
| Hawaii | Honolulu |
| Idaho | Boise |
| Illinois | Springfield |
| Indiana | Indianapolis |
| Iowa | Des Moines |

| | |
|---|---|
| Kansas | Topeka |
| Kentucky | Frankfort |
| Louisiana | Baton Rouge |
| Maine | Augusta |
| Maryland | Annapolis |
| Massachusetts | Boston |
| Michigan | Lansing |
| Minnesota | St. Paul |
| Mississippi | Jackson |
| Missouri | Jefferson City |
| Nevada | Carson City |
| New Hampshire | Concord |
| New Jersey | Trenton |
| New Mexico | Santa Fe |
| New York | Albany |
| North Carolina | Raleigh |
| North Dakota | Bismarck |

| | |
|---|---|
| Ohio | Columbus |
| Oklahoma | Oklahoma City |
| Oregon | Salem |
| Pennsylvania | Harrisburg |
| Rhode Island | Providence |
| South Carolina | Columbia |
| South Dakota | Pierre |
| Tennessee | Nashville |
| Texas | Austin |
| Utah | Salt Lake City |
| Vermont | Montpelier |
| Virginia | Richmond |
| Washington | Olympia |
| West Virginia | Charleston |
| Wisconsin | Madison |
| Wyoming | Cheyenne |

# States and Capitals:

1. Form your group. Begin by asking the question, "What is the capital of New Mexico?" Give hints if needed.
2. If your group is having difficulty with this task, rephrase the question. For example, "Salt Lake City is the capital of which state?" It is often easier to recall the names of states.
3. Multiple choice option: "Austin is the capital city of which state? Is it New York, Ohio, or Texas?"
4. Have you visited or lived in any of these areas?
5. Have you ever visited your state capital?
6. Did you have to memorize the states and capitals in school?

# Book Group/Book Study

**Supplies:** Any book of fiction or non-fiction

**Directions:** Read a few short chapters of any fiction book, or a passage from the Bible. Explore the story by discussing the chapters with a few of the questions below. Don't correct a participant if he or she gives a wrong answer. The goal is to gain confidence in participation and promote conversation.

## Questions for Book Group:

1. Who are the main characters? How many characters can we name at this point? Are they all friends? Are they on the same side or are they rivals

2. What can you tell us about the main characters' personalities? What do we know about the lives they lead?

What are their strengths and weaknesses? What is

important to the main character?

3. What do you think the main conflict will be in this story?

What types of conflicts have we noticed this far?

4. Can we tell at this point, what type of story this will be? Is it

fiction? Do you think it will be a fast-paced story? Is it a love

story? A mystery? A western?

5. How would you describe the setting? Is the setting rural or

urban? Do the characters seem to fit into this setting? Why

or why not?

6. How many characters have we met at this point? Do you

have a favorite? Why? Are there any characters you don't

particularly care for?

7. Have you noticed any props that seem important to the story? Does the protagonist have a particular item that he/she is particularly fond of?

8. Do you think there is any significance in the characters' names?

9. What do you think we will see in the next few chapters? What would you like to see?

# Book Group as Reminisce

Other methods of discussion may include a *reader response* type of dialogue between you and the group. Rather than asking questions, readers are encouraged to share memories of their own lives as they relate to the story.

1. "I can relate to the main character because…"

2. "The protagonist reminds me of…"

3. "The main setting is in Salt Lake. I remember growing up in the city…"

4. "My mother was so much like_____".

5. "Has anyone visited this setting? Does the setting remind you of any place you have been?"

6. "Although I am older than the main character, I recall…"

7. "I envy the way the character handled this conflict because…"

8. "My favorite passage from the book is_____".

9. "I once dealt with the same issue as the main character…"

# Time for Reflection

➢ How is the club interacting?

➢ Do the residents seem to enjoy the story? This is where facial expressions and gestures may be important. Is the story appropriate for the audience? Is it easy to follow?

➢ Is the group providing feedback?

➢ Is the group attentive? If not, are there too many persons in the group? Can the group be divided into two smaller groups?

➢ Is the timing of each reading about right? Too long? Too short?

➢ Are the residents attending the group regularly? Have you lost attendance in the past few weeks? Try visiting with the resident. Perhaps he or she enjoyed the group but could not hear. Maybe she regularly has visitors during group.

# Reading as a Pastime

Was reading an important activity in your family?

What types of books did you read?

How old were you when you learned to read?

Who taught you to read?

Did your parents enjoy reading?

Did you like to read poetry?

Do you remember your favorite authors?

Did you read stories that had a lot of action?

Do you remember any characters from your favorite books?

Did your family own many books? Did you borrow them?

Do you know how much a book cost when you were a kid?

Do you prefer a hardback or paperback?

Do you know that you can now read books on the computer?

How do you think things have changed today?

# The Statue of Liberty

The Statue of Liberty stands in what harbor? (New York Harbor)

The Statue of Liberty is how many feet tall?  (305 feet)

The outside of the Statue of Liberty is made of what metal? (Copper)

The statue represents America's independence from what which country? (Great Britain)

The man who created the sculpture, Frédéric Auguste Bartholdi was from what country? (France)

The famous engineer involved in creating the statue is more famously known in France for designing what tower? (The Eiffel Tower).

What caused leaking in the statue's torch? (Americans decided to add windows to the torch, which leaked and led to deterioration).

Which US President helped to raise money for the statue's reconstruction in the 1980's? (Ronald Reagan)

# Outdoor Adventures

## Can You Guess this Place?

I'm in a place, outdoors along the southern coast of Florida. There is a national park named after this place. Can you guess where? Native Americans called this land *Pa-hay-okee* or "grassy river".

There are over 300 species of birds here. It's part prairie and part jungle. Cypress trees grow here along with orchids, ferns, and saw grass. The location is known for alligators. What is the name of this place? (Everglades)

# Outdoor Adventures

**Can you guess this place?**

  This Brazilian City, located on the Atlantic Coast, is well known for its beautiful scenery and warm temperatures. You won't need to bring a winter coat, as this area lies near the Tropic of Capricorn, and temperatures rarely fall below 50 degrees. The city is a huge tourist attraction hosting more visitors than any other city in South America. The name of the city means, "January River". This place is near the famous beaches of Copacabana and Ipanema.  This city is the site for the 2016 Summer Olympics. (Rio de Janeiro)

# The Declaration of Independence Trivia

- Who wrote the Declaration of Independence? (Thomas Jefferson)

- How many days did it take to write the Declaration of Independence? (17)

- During the revisions of the Declaration of Independence, the men most argued most about what? Was it the about the wording of the document or slavery? (Slavery)

- On what date, was the Declaration of Independence approved by Congress? (July 4, 1776)

# The Declaration of Independence Trivia

- Which two famous men who were involved in the writing of the Declaration of Independence died on the Nation's 50th birthday? (Thomas Jefferson and John Adams on July 4, 1826)

- Who was the first man to sign the Declaration of Independence? (John Hancock)

- During these years, which religious group was not allowed to vote, enter politics, or practice law? (Catholics)

- Many of our founding fathers believed in equality, but owned _____? (Slaves)

# The American Flag

Who sewed the American Flag? (Betsy Ross)

How many stripes does the flag have? (13)

What do these stripes represent? (The 13 original colonies)

How many stars does the flag have? (50)

What do the stars represent? (50 States)

Do the stripes run horizontally or vertically? (Horizontally)

What color are the flag's stripes? (Red and white)

What color is the rectangular shape in the upper corner? (Blue)

What color are the flag's stars? (White)

What are you supposed to do if the flag touches the ground? (Burn it)

What does it mean if the flag is flown up-side down? (It is in distress)

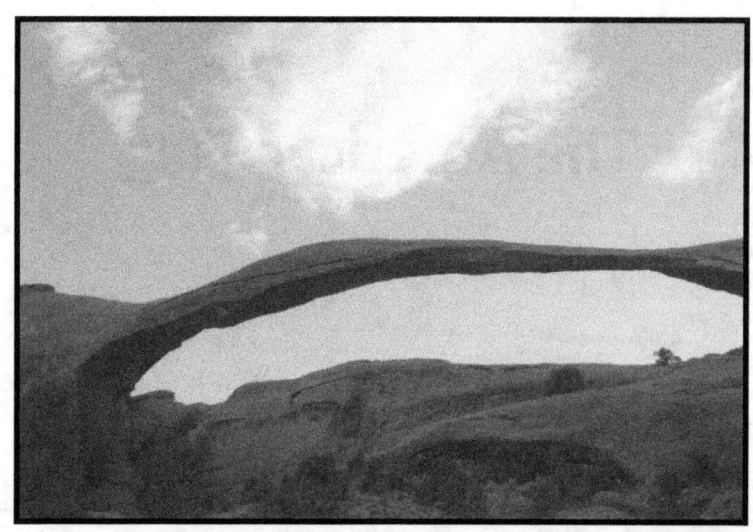

# Can You Guess This National Park?

## Arches National Park

This National Park is located in Southern Utah near the Colorado River. It is well known for its large rock formations. These formations began over 150 million years ago when erosion began shaping the earth into what we know as natural arches. Landscape arch is over 290 feet long, and is the longest natural arch in the world.  One day, erosion will destroy this area's beautiful features in the same way they were created.

# Can You Guess This National Park?

## (Yellowstone National Park)

This national park is located in Montana, Idaho and Wyoming. It is the oldest national park in the world. It is famous for geysers and hot springs. The Grand Canyon and Old Faithful are located here. In 1988 forest fires burned about 45 percent of the park. In this national park, you will see bear cubs, moose, waterfalls and petrified forests. The weather can be a little unpredictable here—don't be surprised to see snow in June! Pioneers often told stories about their visits and explorations of this place, but people often dismissed the stories as tale-tales. Can you guess the name of this national park?

# Niagara Falls

**Can you name this place?**

The place I'm thinking of is located in the Northeast United States and Canada. It draws site-seers from all over the globe. It is well known for its waterfalls which were formed during the last ice age nearly 10,000 years ago. The "falls" are typically perceived to be two separate waterfalls, when in fact, it is actually one large body of cascading water which is divided into two sections— Horseshoe Falls and American Falls. It is the most powerful waterfall in North America, and an important source of hydroelectric power. This landmark is located on the Niagara River.

# Reading Retention

**Memory:** In order to be able to remember and recite information, we usually need to have it presented more than once. It also helps to be able to link new information to what we already know, or to something that is important to us. Try this activity in a small group of five or six people.

**Directions:** Read a short article from the local newspaper or magazine. Ask the group how many facts they can remember. Give no clues at first and allow participants ample time to respond. Read the article again. If the group doesn't seem to remember many facts, start introducing small clues to trigger memory. Read the article a third time. This time ask specific questions relating to the piece.

- What is the article about?
- Who is involved?
- What happened?
- Why is this important to you?

# My Life

## Remembering WWII

*The war changed the lives of many people. Gather a small group and ask them to tell you how the war changed their lives.*

During WWII, I have heard that many things were "rationed". Can you tell me what that means? What types of things were rationed?

How did the war change your family? Did you know someone who served the country?

How did the war change the lives of women?

Were you married before war broke out?

Where were you stationed?

What were "black-outs"?

Today, we have many more sources of information from telephones, internet, TV and radio. How did things differ in war times?

# Remembering WWII

Can you name any of the concentration camps?

Do you know any women who served in the war? What was her role in the war?

How did you hear that the war was over? Do you remember where you were?

How did you celebrate the end of WWII?

Do you remember any books or movies about WWII? Do the movies depict that time period accurately?

Do you have any pictures from that time period?

Did the war shape your values in any way?

If there was one thing you could teach the younger generation about this time in history, what would it be?

# My Life

## Remembering High School

Describe your high school. What was it like?

What were your favorite subjects?

What were your least favorite subjects?

How do you think schools differ today?

Did you learn a second language in school? Can you remember how to say anything in that language?

How did you get back and forth to school?

Do you remember any of your teachers? Did you have a favorite? Did you have any you didn't like?

How many children were in your class? How about in your graduating class?

How did school differ from school today?

How did school prepare you for the rest of your life?

# Reminiscing During Daily Activities

Morning Routine

(Dressing and Grooming)

- Do you remember getting your children ready in the morning?
- What was your morning routine?
- How many children did you have?
- Did you work away from home?

Mealtime

- What is your favorite meal?
- What do you prefer hot food or cereal?
- Who made breakfast in your home?
- Do you like frozen dinners?

Bedtime Routine

- Do you remember getting ready for bed as a kid?
- How many children were in your family?
- Did everyone bathe at night, or certain days of the week?
- Do you prefer going to bed early or late?

# Relaxation Technique

## Visualization

Choose a comfortable place to sit or lie. Start your relaxation activity by telling everyone that this exercise requires complete silence. Prompt your group to close their eyes, and breathe deeply...

Inhale, take a deep breath.

Exhale, let the air out slowly.

*(Repeat 3-4 times)*

Imagine you are sitting in the warm sun on a beach. There are no sounds around you. The rays are warming your entire body. You feel warmth in your limbs and internal organs. You have no pain here. Imagine the scenery as you breathe slowly. What types of things do you see?

Allow the group to image for a short time. After a few minutes, it is time to end the session.

Now, we're about to leave the beach for time being. When you open your eyes, you will feel refreshed and full of energy. One, wake your eyes without opening them. Two, Open your eyes. Three, you are completely awake and full of energy.

# Non-sense Words

**Directions:** Read each word aloud, one at a time. Ask the group what the word makes them think of. There are no wrong answers.

**Example:** If I say the word *Gorgilla,* what does it make you think of? Likely answers may be *gorgeous* or *gorilla.*

## Try This:

Try this group activity around a table and keep pencils and paper handy to encourage people to write, doodle, or sketch as they think.

| | | | |
|---|---|---|---|
| Gorgilla | Beautible | Pibble | Limmer |
| Mustify | Clockpot | Stapron | Shomer |
| Bellavision | Gronnett | Ginafore | Spiffen |
| Frailroad | Seanut | Scruggie | Druggle |
| Hoolhouse | Marfet | Loshay | Mogular |
| Creeple | Barthloom | Glariott | Gangle |
| Demory | Lation | Amerinable | Trainish |
| Delizer | Skwimming | Moonkey | Mediquary |

# Word Association

*Gather a group around a table, or semi-circle. Read each word aloud. Begin the activity by giving a simple introduction or direction, such as, "What does the word _____ (insert word) make you think of?" There are no wrong answers as each person's memory will trigger a different response.*

| | | | |
|---|---|---|---|
| July | Harvest | Animal | Sour |
| Storm | Wish | Angel | Pattern |
| Cookies | Roses | Butter | Fresh |
| Tears | Fuel | Chicken | Smoke |
| Doctor | Lilac | Bleach | Lavender |
| Wedding | Deliver | Spanking | Money |
| Fire | Baking | Wheat | Toy |
| Dustbowl | Wagon | Package | Purchase |
| Photograph | Radio | Telephone | Pet |

# Coloring

## Did You Know?

Feeling stressed? Grab a box of crayons! Research shows that various forms of art—even coloring, can help reduce stress, alleviate pain, and maybe even help you sleep better. When a person colors, paints, or sketches he or she tends to focus only on the artistic task—all other thoughts and distractions disappear. Color therapy, as well as other art therapies, is now being used to help children and adults with diagnosis ranging from anxiety, ADHD, Post-traumatic Stress Disorder, and insomnia.

and sketching can be very therapeutic as well as age-appropriate. The goal is to introduce the activity as such by using a wide selection of coloring pages, as well as a variety of crayons, markers, and colored pencils. Once you have your art supplies on the table, gather residents and read the "Did you know" section aloud.

**Supplies needed:** Various coloring pages from the web, mandalas, or adult coloring books, large pack of crayons, felt-tip markers, or colored-pencils.

Feel free to photocopy and color the design on the following page.

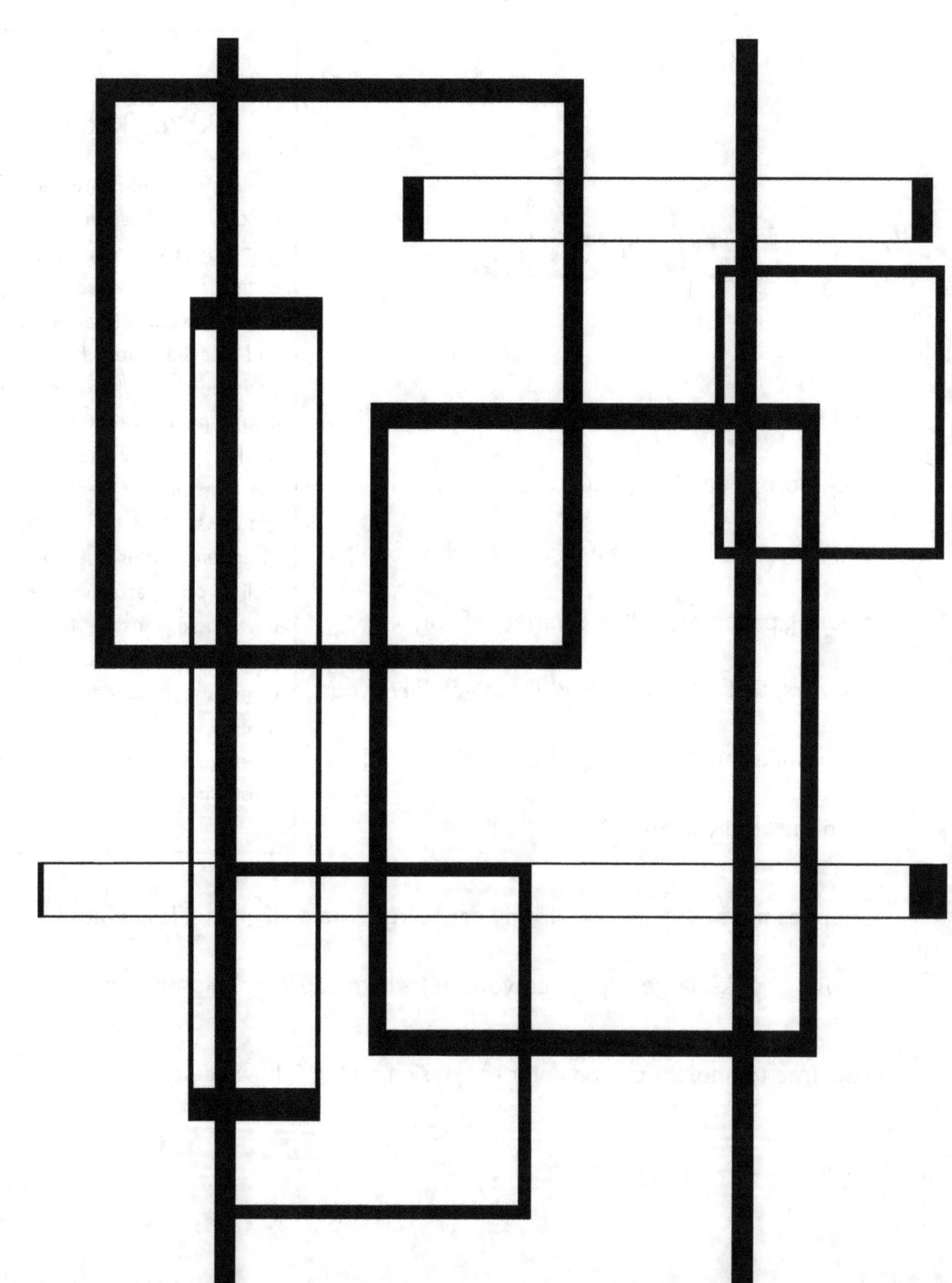

# Things Your Mother Said

If you fall down and break your leg, don't come running to me!

If you keep making that face, it will freeze like that.

Because I said so, that's why.

I have eyes in the back of my head.

How many times do I have to tell you?

If everyone else jumped off a bridge, would you?

Finish your plate. There are children starving in _____.

Be good! Santa Clause is watching!

Go ask your father.

Don't ask why. The answer is no.

Do you think money grows on trees?

Shut the door. We don't live in a barn.

Don't put that in your mouth. You don't know where it's been.

Nobody asked you.

When I was your age...

# Things Your Mother Said

You will eat it, and you will like it.

Don't run with scissors.

Always wear clean underwear in case you get into an accident.

Are your hands broken, or something?

I am not your maid.

Do you think your father and I are made of money?

Get back here when I'm talking to you!

Clean your room! I can't find the floor.

Just wait until your father gets home!

If you can't say anything nice, don't say anything at all.

As long as you live under my roof...

Are you going out in that?

Don't make me come in there!

*Life* isn't fair.

How dumb do you think I am?

# Remembering the One-Room Schoolhouse

Where did you attend school?

Did you attend school in a one-room schoolhouse?

How many children attended your school?

How many other schools were in your area?

Do you remember your teacher?

How did the teacher discipline?

How can you describe the inside of the school?

Were there many other children your age?

Where was the restroom located?

How did you get to school every day?

Did you ever skip school? Were there consequences?

What was your favorite subject?

What was your least favorite subject?

Were there any types of extra-curricular activities?

# Remembering the One-Room Schoolhouse

Did you attend dances, spelling bees, or other social events?

How was the schoolhouse heated?

What types of fuel were used in the heaters?

How many months out of the year was school held?

Where did you get drinking water during the hot months?

Did your school have a playground?

What types of things did you do at recess?

Was the Bible read in school?

Where did the teacher live? Did she stay with the families?

Who paid for the text books?

How did you pass the eighth grade? Did you take a written exam?

Can you remember your school lunches? What did you have to eat?

Did you use a slate or paper and pencils for assignments?

# Remembering the One-Room Schoolhouse

Can you explain what "sweeping compound" is?

What was your earliest memory of school?

Do you remember any games you played in school?

How did you start your school day?

Do you remember when your school was closed?

Is your schoolhouse still standing?

Did school close in bad weather?

What were the most important lessons you learned in school?

Can you tell me what a "box social" is?

Did any of the children speak a language other than English?

What did the girls wear to school? The boys?

Was discipline important in school? Why?

Did you participate in sports?

Do you remember any songs from school?

# Childhood Rhymes

How many of the following rhymes do you remember? Fill in the blanks with your answer.

Little Bo-Peep has lost her _____.

There was an old woman who lived in a _____.

Old Dan Tucker was a mighty _____.

Old Mother Hubbard went to her _____.

Hickory dickory _____.

There was an old woman who swallowed a _____.

One, two, buckle your _____.

# Childhood Rhymes

Mary, Mary, quite contrary. How does your _____?

Rock-a-bye baby, on the _____.

Rain, rain go _____.

Hush little baby, _____.

The itsy-bitsy spider _____.

Ring-a-round the _____.

Here we go round the _____.

Pussy cat, Pussy cat, where have you _____?

Little Boy Blue, go blow your _____.

# What Decade?

The following list of names, terms and phrases are associated with a particular decade. Can you guess the decade?
*Answer: 1920's*

| | |
|---|---|
| Theater | Prohibition |
| Harlem Renaissance | Al Capone |
| Charles Lindbergh | Flapper |
| Blues | Radio |
| Baseball | Movies |
| *The Saturday Evening Post* America | Miss |
| *Spirit of St. Louis* | Tom Mix |
| Sultan of Swat | Censorship |
| Greta Garbo | Jazz |
| Red Grange | Coolidge |
| *The Ten Commandments* | Babe Ruth |

*"I, Too"*

*By Langston Hughes*

*I, too, sing America.*

*I am the darker brother.*

*They send me to eat in the*

*   Kitchen*

*When company comes,*

*But I laugh,*

*And eat well,*

*And grow strong.*

*Tomorrow,*

*I'll be at the table*

*When company comes.*

*Nobody'll dare*

*Say to me,*

*"Eat in the kitchen,"*

*Then.*

*Besides,*

*They'll see how beautiful I am*

*And be ashamed—*

*I, too, am America.*

# At the Market

Grab your local sales advertisements. Give each person a different section. Look at the prices and discuss how prices differ from what they were in the past.

| | |
|---|---|
| 12 oz package of bacon | $2.99 |
| Toothpaste | $1.99 |
| Graham crackers | 2 for $5.00 |
| A can of green beans | $.59 |
| 4 pounds of sugar | $3.00 |
| A box of cereal | $2.99 |
| Lunch meat | 2 for $6 |
| Red peppers | $2.59 per pound |
| A head of cauliflower | $1.99 |
| Whole cantaloupe | 2 for $3.00 |
| A half gallon of milk | $1.50 |
| A loaf of bread | $1.30 |
| Sweet corn | $4.00/doz |
| Jumbo hotdogs | $.99 |
| Peaches | $1.28 per pound |

# Historical Phrases

"I have a dream…"

*Dr. Martin Luther King, Jr.*

"O say can you see, by the dawn's early light"

*The Star-Spangled Banner*

"I pledge allegiance to the flag…"

*The Pledge of Allegiance to the Flag*

"Fourscore and seven years ago…"

*Abraham Lincoln, Gettysburg Address*

"We the people of the United States…"

*The Constitution of the United States of America*

"When in the course of human events…"

*The Declaration of Independence*

# Favorite Things

*Find out more about your group by asking about their favorite things. Pick a phrase from the list.*

What is your favorite _____? Tell us why.

| | | |
|---|---|---|
| Time of day | Month | Day of the week |
| Holiday | Meal | Place you have visited |
| Television show | Hobby | Book or movie |
| Scent | Desert | Junk food |
| Activity | Animal | Place |
| Music | Sport | Outdoor activity |
| Season | Color | Prized possession |

# Groups of Three

If I had three wishes...

Three things I miss the most...

Three things I would want with me on a deserted island...

Three things I wish I could change about the future...

Three things I'd like to bring back from the past...

Three modern conveniences I can do without...

I am most thankful for these three things...

Three things I wish I would have done differently...

Three things I would like to teach younger people...

Three things I would rather be doing...

Three things I procrastinate most about...

Three things that make me happy...

Three things that make me laugh...

# Groups of Three

Three things that bother me the most...

Three things that make me lose my patience...

Three things I never argue about...

Three foods I will never eat...

Three occupations I would never have...

Three things I would never try...

Three ways a person can make me mad...

Three things that should be against the law...

Three things people should not do...

Three things people should not wear...

Three things I would like to try...

# Misplaced

*Read the groups of words below. Which word doesn't belong? Why?*

| | | | |
|---|---|---|---|
| Piano | Orchid | Trumpet | Violin |
| Lamp | Desk | Sofa | Elephant |
| Car | Bus | Truck | Sausage |
| Nurse | TV | Banker | Police |
| Film | Radio | Movie | Blanket |
| Candy | Cake | Sugar | Cat |
| Glass | Tomato | Cup | Mug |
| Femur | Fibula | Tarsal | Greek |
| Peony | Rose | Skunk | Lilly |
| Coffee | Toast | Egg | Spaghetti |

# Book Titles

How many of these book titles can you name? Have you read any of the books on the list? Which were your favorites? Why?

*The Great _____ (Gatsby)*

*The Catcher in the _____ (Rye)*

*The Call of the _____ (Wild)*

*Anne of Green _____ (Gables)*

*Little House on the _____ (Prairie)*

*Gone with the _____ (Wind)*

*Brave New _____ (World)*

*The Cat in the _____ (Hat)*

*Tarzan of the _____ (Apes)*

*The Maltese _____ (Falcon)*

*Winnie the _____ (Pooh)*

# Book Titles

The Sun Also _____ (Rises)

To Kill a _____ (Mockingbird)

Where the Red Fern _____ (Grows)

Lawrence of _____ (Arabia)

A Tale of Two _____ (Cities)

Robinson _____ (Crusoe)

The Adventures of Huckleberry _____ (Finn)

The Three _____ (Musketeers)

The Old Man and the _____ (Sea)

Invisible _____ (Man)

War and _____ (Peace)

# Poetry

*Read three short poems from any book of poetry. You can compose your poem on paper, or a large dry erase board. Start with one line, and ask the residents to add the following line. Keep building your poem until your group feels satisfied with the composition. If you have a singer in the group, you may ask him/her if it would make a good song. Can we put this to music? What would it sound like? You may want to use the following lines to get started.*

I once had a girl...

Walking in the dreary fog...

I met my true love...

Underneath the midnight stars...

A best friend...

My mother once told me...

I learned a lesson...

# Which Decade?

## (1950's)

- ➢ Minimum wage was $.75 per hour.

- ➢ First American satellite was launched.

- ➢ Gas was about $.29 per gallon.

- ➢ Joseph Stalin died.

- ➢ Korean War begins.

- ➢ Dwight D. Eisenhower served two terms as president.

- ➢ Alaska became the 49$^{th}$ state.

- ➢ Hawaii became the 50$^{th}$ state.

- ➢ The Soviet Union launched *Sputnik.*

- ➢ The Cold War begins.

# Money Trivia

- Do you know whose face is on the dollar bill? *(Washington)*

- This president's portrait is on the two dollar bill. *(Jefferson)*

- On the five dollar bill you will find a portrait of which president? *(Abraham Lincoln)*

- Who is the man on the ten dollar bill? *(Hamilton)*

- Whose portrait is on the twenty-dollar bill? *(Jackson)*

- Who is on the fifty dollar bill? *(Ulysses Grant)*

- Can you guess whose portrait is on the one-hundred dollar bill? *(Benjamin Franklin)*

# From the Earth

- Can you guess this mineral? In the middle 1800's, people flocked to California from Europe, South America, and the Eastern United States to "pan" for this mineral. Can you guess what this valuable mineral is? *(Gold)*

- Aluminum is extracted from this mineral. This mineral is found in clay near the surface of the Earth. Can you guess this mineral? *(Bauxite)*

- What mineral is used to make wallboard and *Plaster of Paris? (Gypsum)*

- This mineral, in pure form, is actually very soft. It is mixed with other substances to make it hard. This mineral is used to make cooking utensils, and tools. *(Iron)*

# Opposites

*Say the first word in the list. Ask your resident or group to say the opposite.*

| | | | |
|---|---|---|---|
| Hard | Soft | Bright | Dim |
| Left | Right | Sunny | Cloudy |
| Long | Short | Stop | Go |
| Real | Fake | Right | Wrong |
| End | Beginning | Hot | Cold |
| Enter | Exit | Summer | Winter |
| Good | Evil | Love | Hate |
| Full | Empty | Heat | Ice |

# Opposites

| | | | |
|---|---|---|---|
| Inside | Outside | Top | Bottom |
| Up | Down | Heavy | Light |
| Young | Old | Giant | Dwarf |
| Win | Lose | Tight | Loose |
| Rich | Poor | Work | Play |
| Give | Take | Boy | Girl |
| Live | Die | Lift | Lower |
| Ill | Healthy | Truth | Lie |
| Solid | Liquid | Ugly | Lovely |
| Grow | Shrink | Straight | Crooked |

# Toys & Games of the Past

Rag_____ (doll)

Hula_____ (hoop)

Yo-_____ (yo)

Mr. Potato_____ (Head)

Play-_____ (doh)

Hop_____ (scotch)

Rubber_____ (band) gun

Tic-tac-_____ (toe)

Sock_____ (monkey)

Lincoln_____ (Logs)

Crayola_____ (crayons)

Barbie _____ (Doll)

Jacob's_____ (ladder)

Jump_____ (rope)

Naughts 'n _____ (crosses)

Teddy _____ (bear)

# Backwards Words

*These words are all spelled backwards. Ask your residents to say the correct word.*

Fles _____          Tlem _____

Taeb _____          Balf _____

Erahs _____         Yrt _____

Noom _____          Yad _____

Eerf _____          Uoy _____

Yob_____            Yek _____

Eeb _____           Lla _____

# Backwards Words

Ro _____

Ot _____

Tuc _____

Ni _____

Eil _____

Si _____

Rac _____

Ddo _____

Yal _____

Eyb _____

Ees _____

Rof _____

Sey _____

Llab _____

Baj _____

Ew _____

Toh _____

Rof _____

# Homemade/Handmade

*Can you think of things which are rarely homemade anymore? Why do you think we have lost some of these traditions? Do you know of anyone who still makes any of these items? Can you describe how any of these are made? (Hint: discuss each word one at a time to allow everyone to participate).*

| | | | |
|---|---|---|---|
| Cheese | Bread | Soap | Jam |
| Pickles | Horseradish | Quilts | Clothing |
| Pie | Pillows | Toys | Candles |
| Noodles | Dolls | Custard | Headcheese |
| Bread pudding | Butter | Ice Cream | Cream |
| Rock candy | Furniture | Down pillows | Rugs |

# Which Century

*Can you guess the century in which the following things were invented?*

Tin can, stethoscope, calculator, wrench       (1800's)

Teddy Bear, lie detector, toaster       (1900's)

Hot air balloon, ambulance, steamboat       (1700's)

Typewriter, safety pin, Coca-cola       (1800's)

Bubble gum, photo copier, Atomic bomb       (1900's)

Submarine, piano, soft drink       (1700's)

Toilet paper, machine gun, stapler       (1800's)

Zipper, dynamite, bicycle       (1800's)

# Which Century?

Corn Flakes, crayons, helicopter                         (1900's)

Bifocals, flush toilet                                    (1700's)

Slinky                                                    (1900's)

Sewing machine                                            (1800's)

Pez candy                                                 (1900's)

Parachute, electronic telegraph                          (1700's)

Tea bags, tractor, model-T                               (1900's)

Postage stamp                                            (1800's)

Parachute                                                (1700's)

Fire extinguisher, thermometer                           (1700's)

# America's Firsts Trivia

1. Who was the first president of the United States? (George Washington)

2. In 1636 the first American college was founded. Can you guess the name of the prestigious college? (Harvard)

"I shall never ask, never refuse, nor ever resign an office"

--George Washington

3. The first public school was built in this city also famous for the Tea Party. (Boston)

4. Elizabeth Blackwell was the first woman in this medical profession. Can you guess her position? (Doctor)

5. The first slaves arrived at Jamestown, which is located in what state? (Virginia)

6. The first skyscraper was built in this city in Illinois. (Chicago)

# Har du set den navle I dag?

*Have you seen your belly button today?*

The above phrase is a Danish greeting. How many of your residents speak a foreign language or remember bits and pieces from their parents or grandparents? Does anyone know sign language or Braille? How many of your residents learned Latin in high school? If you have someone who speaks a language, they easily become the "expert". Ask questions while you are in a group. "How do you say, hello? Goodbye? My name is...?"

# Categories

What do the following have in common?

- Tuna, salmon, walleye (types of fish)

- Rye, wheat, white (types of bread)

- Apple, cherry, pear (fruit)

- Oak, elm, spruce (trees)

- Los Angeles, New York, Chicago (major US cities)

- Nile, Amazon, Mississippi (rivers)

- Red, white, blue (colors of the flag)

- Dress, ring, flowers, groom (things a bride has)

- Nickel, penny, dime (change)

- Asia, Africa, North America (continents)

- Atlantic, Pacific, Indian (oceans)

- Moscow, Tokyo, Beijing (capitals or major international cities)

# Which US City

**Las Vegas**

- The name of this US city means, "The Meadows" in Spanish

- It was first discovered by Spanish explorers.

- This city was first a part of Arizona territory.

- It is one of the fastest growing cities in the US.

- The growth of this city is largely attributed to gambling.

- This city is well known for its many wedding chapels,

  casinos, shopping, fine dining and Elvis impersonators.

- It is the most populous city in the state of Nevada.

# Synonyms

*Synonyms are words that have the same, or almost the same meaning. How many synonyms can your group name for the following words?*

| | | |
|---|---|---|
| Turf | Cup | House |
| Plant | Up | Child |
| Walk | Boulder | Path |
| Large | Happy | Laugh |
| Talk | Soft | Community |
| Conflict | Rich | Taunt |
| Rapid | Eat | Construct |
| Start | Small | Good |
| Coat | Slacks | End |

# Sequencing

What holiday comes after Christmas?

Which season comes before spring?

What month comes after March?

What day comes after Saturday?

What meal comes after breakfast?

What season comes after summer?

What month comes after July?

What letter comes after the letter, *M* in the alphabet?

What holiday comes after Easter?

What is the first day of the week?

# Memory Books

**Supplies needed:** Small three-ring binder, stickers, photos, permanent markers, glue, acid-free paper, three-hole punch.

Photocopy the following pages, punch, and insert in binder. Have residents decorate the covers, and insert pictures as they wish. Pictures should be protected in sleeves, or between sheets of acid-free paper.

Copy enough of the daily schedule sheets for two weeks to a month. Remember to check back with your resident frequently to see if more schedule sheets are needed. Don't present this as an assignment that you are checking up on, this is an activity, not a task and should be something the resident enjoys.

Some residents will need assistance with the worksheets. Don't try to fill them all out in one day, but add to them as memories come to the resident.

For those with mild dementia, keep the books on a bedside table for convenience. The books will help a resident remember what he or she has accomplished in the past few days, and assist him in setting new goals and challenges. Include a few sheets of blank paper to give the resident a chance to include drawings, doodles, pictures, or other things he/she may wish to include.

**Benefits:** Improve word-finding skills, encourage creativity, thought organization, short and long-term memory, self-esteem, and fun!

## Daily Schedule

**Today is** _____ **Date** _____

Wake up time _____ Breakfast _____

Exercise _____ Lunch _____

Dinner/Supper _____ Bed _____

An activity I attended today:

_____

_____

_____

Things I would like to do tomorrow:

_____

_____

_____

_____

Upcoming Events/Activities/Appointments:

_____

_____

_____

_____

# About Me

My full name: _____

I was named after: _____

One of the earliest memories of my parents: _____

_____

Five things most important to me: _____

_____

_____

Things I am most proud of: _____

_____

My favorite childhood toys were _____

_____

Something I remember about my siblings: _____

_____

_____

Important things my parents taught me:

_____

_____

My favorite hobbies:

_____

# My Favorites

Use The table below to fill in your favorite things.

| Movies | Foods | Flowers |
|---|---|---|
| Colors | Hobbies | Books |
| People | Animals | Places |
| TV Shows | Activities | Other |

# Timeline of My Life

I was born in _____

I began school in _____

The year I started my first job _____

I got married in the year of _____

I had my first child in _____

I retired in the year of _____

Something exciting happened in the year of _____

The year(s) I remember the most _____

_____

# In the Kitchen

Can you unscramble these words?

1. KSNI

2. LRBNDEE

3. OSVET

4. ATROSTE

5. UPC

6. LEBTA

7. NROCTEU

8. KFOR

| Word Bank |
|-----------|
| Cup |
| Sink |
| Fork |
| Table |
| Counter |
| Blender |
| Stove |
| Toaster |

# Word Find

How many words can you find in the boxes below? Write your answers below the puzzle.

| S | O | B | L |
|---|---|---|---|
| D | E | T | Q |
| K | F | A | N |
| E | R | U | M |

_____

_____

_____

_____

_____

# The Human Body

```
N  Q  S  N  L  Z  M  T  V  M  A  R  R  O  W
I  R  E  B  W  C  J  D  E  E  I  W  V  S  B
C  R  S  L  T  A  L  T  P  M  U  S  C  L  E
F  L  P  C  I  R  P  D  I  O  R  G  A  N  S
I  M  A  E  S  T  A  C  D  E  C  R  S  D  W
B  F  N  Y  S  I  S  K  E  L  E  T  O  N  I
E  K  Y  S  U  L  R  B  R  S  T  V  U  H  L
R  C  S  I  E  A  K  L  M  L  V  R  L  Y  O
S  T  P  N  H  G  X  A  I  L  T  A  M  A  K
U  M  U  U  U  E  Q  J  S  E  Q  P  L  Y  V
I  I  L  S  M  R  Y  R  A  C  H  X  Q  J  R
D  X  S  H  E  A  R  T  T  K  L  I  S  H  Q
A  X  E  Y  R  S  A  E  R  C  N  A  P  M  S
R  C  O  Q  U  S  E  I  D  O  B  I  T  N  A
J  C  P  H  S  F  W  Y  N  E  R  V  E  X  B
```

# The Human Body

## (Word Bank)

| | |
|---|---|
| TISSUE | ANTIBODIES |
| ORGANS | RADIUS |
| NERVE | HUMERUS |
| VALVE | SKELETON |
| HEART | MARROW |
| SINUS | MUSCLE |
| SYNAPSES | FIBERS |
| EPIDERMIS | PANCREAS |
| PULSE | CARTILAGE |
| CELLS | LYMPH |